J Mc Elliott

Polio
'53

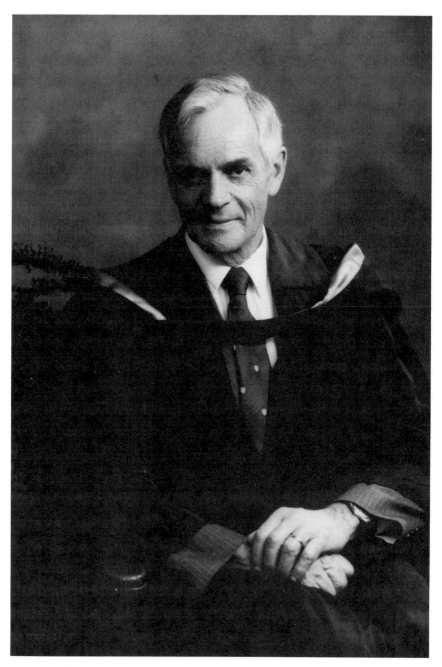

Dr. Russell F. Taylor

A Memorial for Russell Frederick Taylor

Polio '53

by Russell Frederick Taylor, MD

With contributions by
Nelson Nix, MD
J.F. Elliott, MD
B.J. Sproule, MD

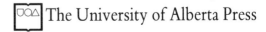 The University of Alberta Press

First published by
The University of Alberta Press
141 Athabasca Hall
Edmonton
Alberta T6G 2E8
1990

The University of Alberta Press gratefully acknowledges the financial
assistance of the Department of Medicine, the University Hospital and the
Royal Alexandra Hospital in the production of this volume.

Canadian Cataloguing in Publication Data

Taylor, R.F. (Russell F.)
A memorial for Russell Frederick Taylor

ISBN 0-88864-230-X

1. Poliomyelitis—Alberta—History.   2. Taylor,
R. F. (Russell F.)   I. Title.   II. Title: Polio '53.
RC181.C22A47 1990   616.8'35'00971231   C90-091530-7

Typesetting by Pièce de Résistance Ltée., Edmonton, Alberta, Canada
Printed by Hignell Printing Ltd., Winnipeg, Manitoba, Canada
Designed by Steve Tate

Contents

ACKNOWLEDGEMENTS

Many people have contributed to the publication of this Memorial. Those particularly deserving of mention are: Diane Chaba, who typed the manuscript into her computer and never complained when yet more editorial changes had to be keyed in; and Margaret Napier, whose organizing skills and enthusiastic hard work behind the scenes were of the greatest value. Others who assisted include the *Edmonton Journal* Archives, brought into action by Mr. Fred Castle, Anne Marie Downie of the Royal Alexandra Hospital, and members of the Taylor family.

Finally, a very big thank you must go to the University of Alberta Hospital, the Royal Alexandra Hospital, and the University of Alberta Faculty of Medicine, without whose moral and financial support this book would never have become a reality.

Russell F. Taylor

Russell Taylor's father, Harry, emigrated from England in 1910 to establish a homestead near Delia, Alberta. He served overseas as a medical corps man during World War I and his background prepared him to assist in emergency first aid situations that occurred in the local farming community.

Evelyn Smith, a VAD (member of Britain's Voluntary Aid Detachment) during the war, met and married Harry Taylor in England shortly before his return to Canada. Russell Frederick, her first child, was born January 29, 1920, on the homestead in the Hand Hills of Alberta. Evelyn Taylor died two years later shortly after the birth of a second son. Russ often wondered if, with proper medical attention, she might have lived. Even as a child he dreamed of becoming a doctor.

His early school years were spent in the one-room Hand Hills school and he later attended school in the town of Delia. The homestead bore the full brunt of the drought and depression years and Russ was able to attend high school in the town of Drumheller only by working for his room and board. A job at the local newspaper, gave him the opportunity to hear Dr. Norman Bethune speak in Drumheller and this rekindled the dream, but reality was work in the coal mines. And reality was eventual enrolment in the Calgary Normal School, where Russ received his teaching certificate in 1940. However, the war interrupted his teaching career before it began and in 1941 he enlisted in the RCAF (Royal Canadian Air Force) transferred to Britain's RAF (Royal Air Force) and served overseas as a navigator.

Active service ended in 1944 with a medical discharge. Two crashes, one in the Canadian Rockies during training and one overseas, had not diminished his love of flying. Russ would eventually become a pilot and instructor with the Edmonton Flying Club. He rejoined the RCAF Auxiliary as a medical officer in 1957 and retired as a Squadron Leader in 1968.

War service earned Russ the opportunity to realize his childhood dream of entering medical school. In 1948 he received a BSc (Honours) in Biochemistry and in 1950 graduated in Medicine from McGill University. In June 1951 he completed his internship at the University of Alberta Hospital in Edmonton. He practiced in Devon, Alberta until June of 1953 when he joined the Allin Clinic in Edmonton. It was during his first year with the Allin Clinic that he was seconded to the Royal Alexandra Hospital to direct the Polio

2

Program. From 1954–62 he continued in general practice with the Allin Clinic.

In 1962 Russ began residency in Internal Medicine at the University of Alberta Hospital and in 1965 became a teaching fellow. After receiving his Fellowship in the Royal College of Physicians and Surgeons in 1966 he joined the Division of Cardiology as an Assistant Professor. He was appointed Associate Professor in June of 1970 and full Professor of Medicine in January 1978.

He became Professor Emeritus in 1985, but continued to serve the Faculty of Medicine of the University of Alberta in various capacities until two months before his death on August 7, 1988.

Foreword

Mary Sullivan

When my father recovered from the operation which revealed he had inoperable cancer, he continued to work at the University Hospital for some months. During that time he asked his long-time friend and colleague, Dr. Garner King, whether there might be some task he ought to undertake for the Department of Medicine and the Faculty in view of the limited time left him. Dad's wish to continue to serve in what he knew to be his last days characterized his devotion to medicine, which was his love and his life.

Dr. Garner King, knowing my father as he did, showed wisdom by making a request of him at that time. Dr. King asked him to write about his experiences during the polio epidemic so that his unique perspective as the director of the Polio Program would not be lost to medical history.

We count it a privilege to be part of this project. At

the same time we are, in some sense, overwhelmed by the wish to do justice to the very dear memory of our father. In terms of the parent, one is ever the child. And from that perspective one looks up, filled with awe of the parent and with the inadequacy of the child self.

We draw courage from the fact that to most of you who will read this, Russ Taylor requires no introduction. You not only knew him, you were part of the greater family of doctors and nurses, of patients and students, who made up the rich fabric of his life.

During the last months of my father's life he received many letters from friends and colleagues. Through this correspondence and through the eulogies prepared by Dr. Rossall and Dr. Blodgett, we have become more aware of the contributions he made.

We know that he filled spaces with his gentleness, his love, and his wisdom. We know that he created spaces with his questions, his courage, and his curiosity. The things people said to my father and about him celebrate who he was. Their tributes say more than I can about Russ Taylor, physician, teacher, and friend.

In an informal sense, my father spent his entire life as a student as he opened himself to experience and sought to understand that experience. Every person, whether friend, colleague, patient, or grandchild presented an opportunity to learn about something. As a colleague said of him, "his enthusiasm for learning about everything was infectious." His friend Ted wrote in the eulogy:

What he wanted to see, and what he barely glimpsed himself was not something we merely knew, but something we should pursue like children with wonder and passion and joy.

Dad was a scholar in the formal sense as well. The subjects of his study apart from medicine, included mathematics and physics, paleontology, history, religion, and philosophy, to list only a few of his interests. And the learning went on in other realms. As an adult he learned to swim, to canoe, and to dance. He was still taking music and French lessons in the last year of his life.

And Dad was a gifted teacher. That may, in fact, have been his greatest sphere of influence. The former Chairman of Medicine, Dr. Donald Wilson, said of his teaching:

> Russ Taylor's contributions to the education of medical students and residents over many years have been simply outstanding. He has served as a wonderful role model of the caring physician to a generation of students.

Many of those former residents and students wrote to thank him for what he gave:

> Your great personal warmth and humanity encouraged me through some very trying times — more than I have ever mentioned. From my time as a cardiology fellow, I remember most your love of teaching and personal interest in each patient. I would like to believe that I am able to emulate you to some extent.

> The highlight of my medical career to date remains the six months I spent as Chief Resident under your guidance. Nothing before or since has matched the sense of fulfilment and excitement of that period. You gave me something much more valuable and difficult to obtain than any medical fact,

a perspective of the whole vast world of medicine, how it all fits together; when to be the clinical investigator, when to be the fellow human being, how to behave towards patients and colleagues and how to keep one's sanity through it all. There is much I still need to learn but any new knowledge will fit into a framework largely of your making.

You always listened sincerely to whoever wanted to talk to you — I am thinking of you as what leaders should be like.

It has always been my hope that I will be able to pursue the understanding of medicine with the vigour that you have demonstrated throughout your medical career — your influence continues to inspire me.

Dad's friend, Dick Rossall, summed it up when he said "teaching was his life blood."

People remembered Russ Taylor for his dedication and sheer hard work. Dr. Rossall said in the eulogy,

To do what he wanted to do would have required a 30-hour day and eight-day weeks. The combination of patient care and teaching consumed him and at times drove other things from his mind.

And from other colleagues came these comments:

I am writing to express my heartfelt thanks for your unflagging support over the years.

Russ always refused to let personal illness interfere with what he considered his obligations personal or professional.

I am especially remembering your passion for looking after the patients and the house-staff from the early morning till late nights.

And my father is remembered for his humanity. Ted Blodgett said it best:

What do we love in Russ? We love that love we all divined. This is why he became the best of doctors. Because he understood profoundly that the illness was natural, and that we as people were so much more important than our afflictions.

Other friends wrote to him:

The highest expression of civilization is not in its art, but the supreme tenderness that people are strong enough to feel and show toward one another. When I think of this remark, you come to mind, Russ. You are an example of all that is fine, generous and courageous.

And of him,

The world is a bit better place because he spent some time here. I hope personally to be able to go on with my life with at least a small bit of the great intelligence, devotion and courage that made Russ, to me, absolutely unique.

Patients wrote to him:

Dr. Taylor, you are truly a godsend and your compassion will forever live in our hearts.

I always felt secure in your hands.

And of him,

I will always be grateful for the long hours he put in with us polios at the Alex, as well as the love and understanding he gave when we desperately needed it.

When he himself was feeling so terribly sick, he asked me how I was and really cared to hear the answer and tried to visit with me — he gave of himself to people through his gentle smile, his sparkling eyes and his quiet ways.

And nurses remembered him,

His humility and kindness were experienced by many. He gave of himself willingly and took on the extras that others were unwilling to do.

His concern for patients and nurses was recognized by everyone.

Dr. Rossall referred in the eulogy to my father's humility. And, in fact, Russ was not aware of the extent of his contribution. He answered a colleague's letter in the last weeks of his life saying:

I often feel diffident about my years at the school — no major research, not even very well informed in lots of areas. These thoughts are persistent and troublesome when there is to be no chance to make any further contributions or retributions.

He was likewise overwhelmed by the ceremony in which his colleagues honoured him for his contributions to the University Hospital. So moved was he by Dr. King's remarks and by the outpouring of respect and affection from his colleagues, that he said he doubted he would be able to sleep that night.

It is appropriate that the polio monograph, apart from its importance in medical literature, is presented here as a memorial tribute to a great physician, teacher, and friend, for the epidemic was an event in my father's life and a period of his life which may indeed have marked him in some special way. The demands of the epidemic on medical personnel, the courage of the patients, the tragedies suffered by the families, and the limitations of medicine in the face of such suffering, no doubt left deep impressions. Perhaps that time had much to do with the making of the physician and the man who emerged in the years that followed.

Dr. Rossall referred to that time in the eulogy he delivered at my father's funeral:

> Russ made an indelible mark on the medical community of Edmonton in the mid 1950s by his incredible and dedicated efforts during the last poliomyelitis epidemic. He literally lived in the Royal Alexandra Hospital with his patients for almost eighteen months and the community owed much to him for that. This is part of the legend.

When Dr. Nelson Nix wrote to my father in response to the polio monograph he said,

> The thing that you 'typically' neglected was your own energetic, thoughtful, innovative leadership which you used to stimulate and encourage the rest of us.

This is true, even to the point that my father wrote much of the monograph in this volume in the third person.

The monograph invites the reader to be reflective, to raise questions, and to seek understanding. This, too, is typical of Dad. In this way he continues to teach us by charging us to probe matters with intellectual and human integrity.

As Russ Taylor's children, my brothers and I think it fitting that our father's achievements and contributions be celebrated. We are grateful to Dr. Garner King for his tenacious pursuit of this publication, and to Dr. Nelson Nix, Dr. Frank Elliott, and Dr. Brian Sproule for their work included here. We are grateful to all the people who were part of the satisfaction and fullness of Russ Taylor's life.

We remember with deep appreciation the surgeons, the physicians, and the nurses who personally cared for Dad in the last year of his life. And we remember with tender gratitude those students, colleagues, patients, and friends who let Dad know, while he was alive, that he made a difference with his life, to theirs. And finally, we extend our love and gratitude to his wife Cora for her steadfast devotion.

MARY SULLIVAN
KEN TAYLOR
JIM TAYLOR
TERRY TAYLOR

CHAPTER ONE

Polio 1953

Russell F. Taylor, M.D.

Introduction

The post-war epidemic of poliomyelitis, which for five years had been making its way west from Austral-Asia, reached Edmonton in the spring of 1953.

It was as if this vibrant, optimistic city had been smitten by a medieval plague; it engendered the same fear and helplessness. Arbitrary and insidious, it struck all ages and conditions, sweeping its victims from buoyant health to paralysis and death within a week.

Like war and like plague, it left its mark on three generations.

This is a reflection on that time.

Infantile Paralysis

During the, '20s and, '30s infantile paralysis was familiar to Albertans. It occurred almost every summer and sometimes there were enough cases for it to be called "epidemic." People were counselled not to "visit about," and to go to town only when necessary. There was particular anxiety about water, and local swimming holes were to be avoided.

Children with various degrees of disability were not uncommon. It was the time of FDR and the March of Dimes.

By 1930 enough children with residual deformity had accumulated to justify the construction of a cottage rehabilitation hospital on the grounds of the University of Alberta Hospital (the Provincial Special Unit).

Although there is no way to establish the fact, it seemed that not many children died of infantile paralysis in those years. Terms like "bulbar" and "respiratory poliomyelitis" were not current.

Polio with respiratory muscle paralysis, however, must have been experienced elsewhere, because in 1927 the British automagnate, Lord Nuffield, designed, built, and then donated an iron lung to each major municipal hospital in the British Empire, including the Royal Alexandra (RAH). An Alex alumnus remembers that as a young scarlet fever patient she saw this machine suitably shrouded and tucked into a corner somewhere in Isolation. It had an air of mystery and menace about it that she would have cause to recall twenty-five years later.

Epidemics of any infectious disease always raise interesting questions even when the organism and vector are known. Polio is an enteric virus infection occurring by hand to mouth transmission of fecal material. It might have been true that the incidence of

14

infantile paralysis was higher in cities and large towns where there was a shared water and milk supply, but cases appeared to be widely and evenly scattered in rural areas. How did it spread?

Epidemics of another enteric infection — typhoid fever — were also common in those years, but these were local and must have centered about a food handler in the family or in the camp, a distribution quite unlike infantile paralysis.

It has been said that most children in pre-war years were infected and rendered immune (unhygienic living conditions?) and that improved hygiene during and after the war allowed a generation to grow into adulthood without immunity. There are problems with this simple proposition. If improvement in sanitation had resulted in a large non-immune population, where did this system break down in 1953? To those on the ground that year there was no apparent pattern. It seemed that once the disease touched down the whole province lit up like an old-fashioned switchboard. Although the case load was heaviest in the cities and larger towns, the disease did not seem to radiate out from any particular place. Somehow the virus found its way into the most remote areas and even up into the far north.

The RAH Experience

Most cases of infection with the polio virus are sub-clinical so the total incidence in 1953 can never be known. The term "polio epidemic" applies most particularly to the unprecedented number of patients with severe generalized paralysis, respiratory paralysis, and the often lethal bulbar form of the disease.

No class or age was spared, but it seemed to be particularly cruel to a generation of young adults. After a short silent incubation period, victims developed a headache, followed by rapidly progressive paralysis and sometimes death within three or four days.

The impact on the community was enormous. At least five nurses were among the victims and two of them died. (Miraculously none of these were from the polio ward!) One doctor nearly died and another was left hemiplegic. A new bride died. Another survived and eventually went home to spend the rest of her life on a ventilator. A lawyer and his wife were both in iron lungs at the same time. This man and two other lawyers died. There were children—a two-year-old girl, some school children, and some teenagers. Three teachers were admitted during the summer of 1953. The litany goes on to a total of 112 cases treated in iron lungs between the spring of 1953 and the fall of 1955. On one day in late November 1953 there was a total of fifty-five patients in the Isolation Hospital, thirty-three of them on respirators attended by eighty-five nurses, and eight doctors!

Poliomyelitis was a reportable disease and it was inevitable that the RAH Isolation Hospital would become the referral centre for Edmonton and northern Alberta. By 1953 this hospital, which had been opened in 1924, was already becoming obsolete, its staff reduced to a few senior nurses. It had no permanent medical staff and only three iron lungs, including the old Nuffield iron coffin, a March of Dimes Drinker–Collins, and one other. Now it was to be confronted with a greater task than any hospital had ever faced in the province's history.

As each patient arrived there was a brief examination, spinal tap, and then triage—home, admit for observation, or admit for ventilation.

Respiratory paralysis was usually progressive and often required at least temporary ventilation support. Under the best circumstances a patient was promptly stabilized in the iron lung without intubation or tracheostomy, but much more commonly, either because there was not enough time or because a lung was not immediately available, it was necessary to intubate and perform an emergency tracheostomy. Once this was accomplished mechanical respiration could be continued with an anesthetic handbag. "Bagging" became second nature to all attendants, lay and professional alike. The need to perform this procedure assumed the highest priority. The first practical step to meet the emerging challenge was taken by Dr. Nelson Nix, then an anesthetist on the staff of the RAH. He asked for a leave of absence to work full time at the Isolation Hospital. Through his operating room experience with intubation and supported ventilation, he was able to provide crucial respiratory support and eventually train others for the same role. Dr. Nix was joined by Dr.R.F. Taylor who had three adult patients admitted to respirators in as many days, two of whom died. Taylor was seconded

17

to the RAH by the Allin Clinic and left immediately to visit a chronic polio unit in Minneapolis for familiarization with the operation of iron lungs.

During this time a committee was struck and put in charge of the polio operation at the RAH Isolation. Among several other members, the committee included Nix and Taylor, Dr. Don Easton (the Medical Superintendent), and Miss Ida Johnson (Matron).

The first priority was to obtain respirators. By 1953 iron lungs were available from previous epidemics elsewhere, but there were never enough locally. Fortunately the Edmonton based RCAF Search and Rescue Squadron co-operated fully with the committee not just in transporting lungs, but also in transporting patients. During the first summer and into fall, there were several tense occasions during which patients became progressively more paralysed while a DC3 was droning its way home with iron lungs on board.

There was an urgent need for nurses. Ida Johnson and the senior Isolation staff were soon completely occupied in recruiting and training new nurses. There was a generous response to the call for volunteers — a portent of how the whole community would eventually rally to the hospital's aid.

Nurses came from other wards in the Alex, from other hospitals, from industry, and from the Military. Many of these volunteers had to continue their regular employment, working the Isolation Hospital into their off time. Overtime and double shifts were the rule and there was no extra compensation.

In addition to nurses, more doctors were urgently needed. The medical problems encountered by a completely paralysed, very ill patient in an iron lung were enormous. These were met by volunteer help from the medical community. Dr. Frank Elliot, a senior specialist in Internal Medicine at the University Hospital, began to spend all of his time on Isolation helping to sort out metabolic and other general medical problems. Dr.Ted Aaron, whose post-graduate training included a year of pulmonary medicine, was also contributing a major part of his time to the unit. Dr. Rice, at that time Professor of Physiology in the Faculty of Medicine, brought help and advice in the area of respiratory physiology, and Dr. Ken Clark made himself available on call for the performance of emergency tracheostomies. An unprecedented phenomenon occurred when the majority of practising physicians in Edmonton, working with the Edmonton Academy of Medicine, established a volunteer roster; because of this there were several physicians present on the polio wards at all times. When these physicians were not engaged in medical procedures, they worked alongside other volunteers moving aching limbs, applying cloths to feverish foreheads, reading to patients, or just visiting. None of the physicians, either on the committee or among the local practitioners, received any remuneration. Finally there was a large and faithful number of lay volunteers — people who served as runners, readers, visitors, and general comforters. Particularly remembered was Ross McBain and his wife, who regularly presented movies

19

and slide shows throughout those long months.

There was also need for money; a fund to put at the disposal of the committee for exigencies, the expenses not covered in institutional budgets. This fund was established by subterfuge. The committee suggested that the provincial government be asked to appoint a director at a salary of $1,000 per month and Dr. Taylor was proposed for the post. Such was the temper of the times that the government accepted this proposal forthwith. Since Taylor was already receiving support from the Allin Clinic, his government salary was diverted to a Polio Fund throughout the nine months of the agreement. When the epidemic was over and the patients transferred from the RAH to the UAH (University of Alberta Hospital), a small sum still in this fund was contributed to the Polio Foundation.

And so the Alex, like a nation at war, began to cope and gain experience.

In the beginning, doctors sometimes delayed too long before committing a patient to the iron lung but as the procedure became less threatening, ventilation was started earlier — a fact that allowed patients to adjust before the onset of total paralysis. Once patients had been placed in the lung, technical questions arose — how much positive or negative pressure, what rate to set, and the often emotional issue of how and when to begin the process of weaning the patient off mechanical support. Electrolyte and acid base imbalance was common, management empirical, corrections often precipitated further metabolic imbalance.

There was preoccupation and uncertainty about the place of tracheostomy. This operation may have created more problems than it solved. Nurses and doctors alike were unfamiliar with tracheobronchial hygiene, nebulization was primitive and each "trach" brought in its wake a nightmare of "plugs" — hard excrescences of blood and mucus that formed and reformed in the trachea and mainstem bronchi. So universal was this complication that the regular staff became quite expert at emergency bronchoscopy and forceps removal of inspissated debris. Ordinary bedside nursing was enormously complicated for patients enclosed in the steel tank. Ironically the only treatment for paralytic polio was physiotherapy and the application of hot packs, impossible to do without opening the iron lung. Again, it was the anesthetists who came to the rescue by training attendants to ventilate by hand — "bagging" — a technique which permitted them to open the iron lung at any time and for as long as needed.

At year's end, most of the major problems had been encountered and a routine established. Ventilator patients occupied two floors of the hospital. There were iron lungs down each side of the ward, huffing and wheezing with remorseless regularity, each surrounded by ancillary equipment — suction apparatus, tanks of O_2, or compressed air. The patients were paralysed and speechless, often terrified because they were unable to communicate. To indicate alarm, patients learned to cluck their tongue against the roof of the mouth— clucking that had to be loud enough to summon help

21

over the noise and confusion of the ward before losing consciousness.

Like any mechanism, iron lungs could and did fail — a leak might occur, or a motor stop. When this happened, manual operation of the lung had to be instituted immediately. Ed Adams, one of the lay volunteers, using the resources of Dominion Instruments, designed a red warning light which was activated if negative pressure was lost for more than one cycle. The presence of this backup alarm was a comfort to staff and patients alike.

Though iron lungs could be operated manually if there was a power failure, it was recognized that an auxiliary power unit should be installed but this was not accomplished until late in the epidemic. On the night of November 20, 1953, Edmonton had a freak electrical storm, causing a power failure in the RAH sector of the city. The nineteen respirators going at that time sighed to a stop. As soon as the lights went down in the nurses residence, student nurses knew instinctively what to do and came running through the wind and rain to the Isolation Hospital.

Ida Johnson called it "my thrill of a lifetime in nursing." She wrote "when I arrived on isolation, I found all of the lungs being manned by student nurses helping the staff on duty. They were in blue jeans, slacks, hair curlers — just as they were when the lights went out in the residence. What a lifesaver they were and what a blessing to the patients' state of mind."

With Alberta, the global postwar polio epidemic ended. During its five year existence, new types of

22

respirators had been developed — most of which eventually found their way to the RAH Isolation — direct positive pressure devices, chest cuirasses, rocking beds. With Dr. Rice's assistance, staff developed their own techniques for physiotherapy, attaching a vacuum cleaner to the lung to give "a good deep breath" followed by the sudden opening of a hand port allowing atmospheric pressure to crash-in on the patient's chest.

By the fall of 1954, the Isolation Hospital had become a Chronic Respiratory Unit. Patients with even the most severe paralysis were being nursed outside of the respirator using the technique of hand bagging. (Patients were usually more comfortable with this method than any other form of ventilation and recognized the good and bad baggers!). In 1955 all remaining cases were transferred to the University Hospital.

The RAH Isolation Hospital was then closed forever.

St. Mary's Ward

From September 1953 until the fall of 1957, the Edmonton General was heavily committed to the care of paralytic and respiratory polio. Most patients came to St.Mary's Ward on transfer from the Alex, but some were admitted directly from the community. One of the first such cases was a boy who had been maintained in a respirator at the Camrose Hospital for six weeks. He had been successfully stabilized under the care of Dr. McGinnis but the old iron lung could not be maintained; still in his lung and connected to a portable generator, this boy was brought by transport van to St.Mary's Ward.

The Edmonton General had just transferred a TB ward to the Aberhart; plans to open a new medical ward were put on hold and St. Mary's was turned over to the polio program.

By 1957 more than seventy-five severely paralysed polio patients had passed through this ward. Many of these required respiratory support, at one time fourteen patients were in iron lungs and seven of them still were at the time of transfer.

Polio survivors may remember the Alex with gratitude, but they remember St. Mary's with affection. This is partly because at that time the Edmonton General was still more a "private" than a "public" hospital, and medical and nursing volunteers were drawn from its own staff. But more importantly, it was due to the dedication of Sister Superior (Bernadette Bezaire) who came to the General in 1953 from Saskatoon where she had gained experience with respiratory patients, and also to the similar dedication of Lillian Hope, Charge Nurse on St. Mary's ward. Both of these nurses were deeply moved by the plight of polio patients and their dedication to the relief of suffering was palpable. (Mrs. Hope's husband raised enough money from his business associates to buy a Coffalator, a device to assist coughing, for the ward. This useful adjunct was shared between St. Mary's and the RAH.)

It was not until 1957 that the last iron lung was

transferred from the General Hospital to the University Hospital, closing one more chapter in the polio saga.

Epilogue

Polio and the Pest House

Contagion and the fear of contagion are as old as recorded history. Canada's first hospital, which opened in 1639, was a Smallpox Hospital. Generations of Canadians were familiar with "quarantine" and "fumigation." School boys regaled each other with stories about a leper train that sped across Canada usually carrying a single leper to some remote leper colony. As in most myths, it always travelled at night! The modern approach to contagion owes much to the establishment of TB sanatoria and the proven efficacy of face masks and hand washing; it has been suggested that even the common cold is transmitted by hand. A recent review in the *Annals of Internal Medicine* concludes that terms like quarantine and isolation should apply to body secretions and not to patients with infections.

Looking back to 1953, one can see that the time was

already approaching when isolation hospitals and sanatoria would close, but in 1953 none of these reassuring notions were current. The Isolation Hospital was regarded as a high-risk environment. The medical staff, the nurses, and lay volunteers who worked there were more than ordinarily careful about masks, gowns, booties, and about hand washings and showers; there was an irregular use of gamma globulin but none of these items reduced the ambient anxiety.

Work in the Isolation Hospital was performed in spite of the perceived risk and in spite of fear.

There is no way now of deciding whether attendants and their families were at increased risk. One of Dr. Nix's children had a mild case. A physician continued to work through a brief febrile illness and subsequently noticed a slight limp. The husband of a ventilator case, himself a tireless volunteer, developed the disease and died. The study of one patient who was a young boy at the time and is now a chronic respirator patient at the Aberhart exemplifies both of these terrors. He spent many months full time in an iron lung and was gradually advanced to other forms of mechanical support including a rocking bed, but always along the way he was encouraged to "breathe on your own." One day a doctor and a nurse decided to give him a treat and take him for a car ride. He still remembers the sheer terror invoked by his very real air hunger and the reassurance of the doctor and the nurse not to worry — his lips weren't blue! There were varying degrees of the same kind of "positive thinking" throughout the polio community.

A great deal of experience has been gained over more than half a century, with surgery to improve function following infantile paralysis and poliomyelitis, and there seems to have been a steady profitable development in this area up to the present time. Whether or not the manipulation of paralysed limbs and the application of hot packs was equally useful is very much in doubt, but what is not in doubt is the unhappy memories polio survivors have of these procedures.

Personal Postscript

My involvement in the 1953 polio epidemic was involuntary — as it must have been for others. One was just swept into the mainstream of events. I best remember the loneliness I felt confronting bulbar polio with a Royal Lifesaving Diploma in artificial respiration! And that loneliness grew. Returning from a few days at the Sister Kenny Institute, where I was to have acquired some special knowledge and skill, I knew, in fact, I had not become better equipped,only more alarmed!

In those first difficult days I was further disconcerted when the *Edmonton Journal* published a front page story announcing my appointment as Polio Director at the princely salary of $1,000 per month. The truth behind the headlines was that I wasn't a director in any operative sense and that the salary had been negotiated to give us an exigency fund.

Whitehead said that a man matures only if he has confronted the cosmos alone. Before the year was out, I had discovered what it felt like to be able to cope with most exigencies in an intensive care environment, and though the skills have since diminished, the attitude has persisted.

By early November 1953, even though the numbers were increasing, most of us felt that we had taken the measure of the epidemic, but for me the greatest single tragedy still lay ahead.

Late in that month — I think it was November 20 — we were consulting with doctors in Grande Prairie on a case of what seemed to be quite rapidly progressive respiratory paralysis. We had suggested that the patient be taken to the OR (operating room) and intubated while we mobilized Search and Rescue to pick him up.

Dr. Aaron, who was in charge of the unit on that day, was contacted by the RCAF who told him that a single engine Cessna had already left Grande Prairie piloted by Gordon MacDonald, with Dr. Don Wilson and his patient on board and that this plane was now overdue. They never did arrive and the wreckage was not found for many months.

All three were young men with families; it exemplifies the kind of reactive behaviour we all exhibited when confronted with these terrified patients and their families.

The patient could have been supported with hand ventilation. The RCAF would then have transported him in an iron lung. The Cessna pilot was experienced and had radio equipment to fly the range. He had done this many times before but, apparently, for some inexplicable reason, tried to descend and fly visually. I have always felt that one of us should have sensed the potential for panic and had the Air Force fly us up to the Grande Prairie Hospital. (The air ambulance still had to wait another decade!)

Finally I want to record how the polio experience at the RAH saved the life of a boy with tetanus. One Sunday in the spring of 1955, Larry Howard, then six years old, stepped on a nail in his father's barn and by Thursday he was in the Royal Alexandra Hospital exhibiting tetanic convulsions. Since respiratory paralysis no longer held any particular terror for me there was no question that he should be treated with curare and put on a ventilator.

With the help of Dr. Gain and the loan of a small positive pressure ventilator from the UAH Anesthesia Department, we were able to control his tetanus and ventilate him for the next twenty days. Dr. Ken Miller and I alternated twelve hour shifts in classical one-on-one ICU fashion and the boy recovered completely.

We later discovered that no case of survival with such a short incubation period had been reported and it was a year or two before any case reports began to appear of patients treated with curarization for this disease.

CHAPTER TWO

Memories of a Personal Confrontation With Poliomyelitis

Nelson Nix, MD

During my years in medical school and internship, "Infantile Paralysis" did not seem to have a high profile. It chiefly affected a few small children, rarely adults. The majority of cases displayed temporary or permanent paralysis of arms, legs, or both. In a small number, breathing was involved. The textbook (1939) that I read recommended that "the child is best treated in the home." Quinine was said to be beneficial in controlling the disease. For respiratory paralysis, there was "artificial respiration and inhalations of oxygen, and these usually fail." Orthopedic corrective measures were developed and in many cases rehabilitation was successful.

As a young teenager in the late 1920s, I did become aware of sporadic outbreaks of polio that occurred in late summer but ended with the first heavy frosts. The return of us children to school was sometimes delayed until October.

In 1941 I was employed as a physician by the Alberta Travelling Clinic from May to August. The last four or five weeks of the planned clinics in outlying rural communities were cancelled. There was general agreement that assemblies of children during polio epidemics were unwise. Furthermore, it was felt that recent tonsillectomies (which we were doing) could render a child more susceptible to the disease. During my further post-graduate training and four years of military service in Canada and Europe, I had no experience with patients in the acute phases of poliomyelitis.

In 1952 we were aware of a serious epidemic of polio in the midwest of the United States and in southern Manitoba. There was an increase of cases in Alberta. By July 1953 a major outbreak in the Edmonton area appeared. Dr. Frank Woodman, a physician from Westlock, Alberta was stricken by polio and did not survive. The gravity of the situation became more apparent. The patients from central and northern Alberta were treated as usual in the Isolation Unit of the Royal Alexandra Hospital.

Late in August, our two-year old daughter dragged a foot for a day or two. She recovered and no investigation was done. But about a week or so later, her six-year-old brother was sent to the Isolation Hospital with paralysis of the throat muscles, diagnosed as poliomyelitis. If we had known then what we were to learn just a few weeks later, the boy probably would have had a tracheostomy. Fortunately, however, his condition did not progress and he was sent home in two weeks to convalesce under the capable care of his mother. The minor swallowing and speech defects disappeared within a year.

Being a staff doctor at the Royal Alexandra Hospital, I was able to visit my son several times a day. As an anaesthetist I was naturally disturbed to observe that there were patients in the open ward who had various degrees of respiratory insufficiency and distress. The nurses and interns appeared to have a heavy responsibility in respect to assessment of the changing status of some patients, and for decisions for much more active care. To me it seemed that in the development of the early effects of respiratory polio there was insufficient knowledge and technique available for resuscitation and on-going support. It did not look as though there were proper plans or trained staff prepared and ready to act. The important thing seemed to be to make the diagnosis, assembling the clinical picture. In retrospect there was probably too much reliance on the spinal fluid test and too little diligence for early, continuous observation and support.

33

After our son returned home, I went to a meeting in Seattle to hear a paper and discussion on how anaesthetists could help in the management and support of patients with acute poliomyelitis, especially those whose breathing was affected. Back in Edmonton, I became involved with the growing number of patients with respiratory problems. It began with being called from the operating room or home to see new admissions with blue lips and fingernails. With the insertion of a breathing tube and pushing oxygen-enriched air into the lungs, the crisis would be averted but not ended. Decisions were required as to the need for a tracheostomy and for sustained artificial respiration by mechanical means. Anaesthetics for tracheostomies in the little operating room were needed, as well as coaching the nursing and resident medical staff on the use of "iron lungs" or respirators.

In this new epidemic, a large number of those afflicted suffered from involvement of the brain stem, causing paralysis of the muscles needed for breathing. The majority of these were young adults.

A whole new system was necessary, without the luxury of a prolonged phasing-in period. The patient with acute poliomyelitis who began to suffer from respiratory distress required the same degree of continuous observation, monitoring, and assistance as was provided to anyone lying on an operating table under general anaesthesia. This called for close, knowledgeable management of the respirator, in respect to its rate, stroke volume, and pressure of the air in the tank. With the benefit of hindsight, it appeared that the medical and nursing staff previously had too little experience in the field of respiratory insufficiency or failure, let alone the on-going management of long-term artificial respiration. Capable medical staff were required on site around the clock, not just for visits once or twice a day.

Dr. Russell Taylor, in family practice with the Allin Clinic, in the autumn of 1953 admitted to the Isolation Hospital three critically ill victims of polio. He stayed with them, wanting to provide every possible help and to consider the new approach that had been obtained at the Seattle workshop. He enthusiastically agreed with the co-operative effort and wanted to work full time with me. Our patient load built up quickly. Dr. J. Frank Elliott left most of his practice at the University Hospital and provided further expertise as an internist. In addition, his uncounted shifts of night duty provided a relief to the previous every-other-night routine. Frank's presence also provided an additional medical specialist to add to those on call. Many other staff members and residents and practitioners from across the city were helping when they were able to do so.

An unusual situation was appearing. Our respirator patients were becoming stabilized, many were surviving, and there was, for almost the first time, reasonable hope. But the only respirators in central Alberta were now in use. Dr. Don Easton was the Royal Alex Medical Superintendent and he used his war-time connections to produce load after load of the bulky machines from Winnipeg and the east. This was done within short hours, courtesy of Search and Rescue pilots of the RCAF.

Although we were encouraged by successes, there were heart-breaking frustrations and defeats. In mid-October 1953 Russell Taylor offered to go to Minneapolis University Hospital, the Kenny Institute, and to Winnipeg, where there had been serious epidemics the previous year. I encouraged and helped him to go. I gave him the names of doctors who had developed some of the newer treatment methods discussed in Seattle. Russell was away a couple of weeks but wrote to me after a few days to pass on "some things that should not wait my return." This included news of an improved respirator which could be used on a hospital bed rather than the unpleasant tank. There was also useful advice on treatment of fever, and some helpful biochemistry tests.

On his return, Russell was tireless in coaching, teaching, and encouraging the staff, the patients, and their families. A retired nurse recalls to this day the instruction classes he gave to new groups of RNs (registered nurses) in the management of respirators. This included placing the nurses in a tank to experience to some degree, the intense emotions of a helpless patient.

An interesting situation initially occurred among some of the medical practitioners in the hospital and the city. The traditional pattern had been that a patient's own doctor would admit to the Isolation Hospital, write the orders and supervise the treatment, using consultants if required. The concept of turning over one's patient to a team of strangers was a shock to some but a welcome relief to others. The hostility to the new method was fortunately short-lived and was replaced by co-operation.

It had been realized quite early by the Royal Alex medical staff that a "Polio Committee" was required. Dr. D.B. Leitch was head of the Department of Pediatrics and he was asked to chair the committee. Other members, who included Dr. Easton and Miss Ida Johnson the Superintendent of Nurses, were the volunteer doctors who were working night and day in the polio wards.

A short while later the committee appointed Dr. Russell Taylor director of the unit. He was a natural, obvious choice, not only because of his leadership skill, but also because of his excellent clinical ability and warm personality. He played a key role in what was to be the biggest medical emergency in the history of Edmonton and central Alberta.

The hospital administration and supporting staffs responded to the new demands with speed and dedication. Ida Johnson, as usual, was proficient in providing the high level of nursing staff required, from volunteers across the city, and from other hospitals and towns.

Generous credit is due to Drs. Douglas Leitch and James Calder and their colleagues, and certainly their staff of dedicated nurses headed by Misses Jean Boyd,

Dorothy Jenner, Sena ("Ma") Thompson, and Violet Chapman. These people had struggled with poliomyelitis, typhoid fever, scarlet fever, diphtheria, tuberculosis, and other dreaded infectious diseases in the three-storey Isolation Hospital. This unit of the Royal Alexandra Hospital had served central and northern Alberta with distinction over many decades.

Dr. Sandy Summerville, Deputy Minister of Health, helped to supply doctors and nurses from the health units and armed forces, as well as ambulances and aircraft to ferry critical patients from rural areas. In November, the provincial government announced plans to provide a "Polio Wing" for the on-going care of the disabled survivors of the epidemic.

The many "imported" nurses, the recent graduates, and the supervisors learned quickly. In their selfless, dependable way they delivered superb care to the patients, including working through the portholes of the tanks with attention to pressure points, medications, catheters, and intravenous drips. Resident doctors and practitioners also became accustomed to providing positive-pressure breathing using a face mask and bag with oxygen. This was necessary at intervals during the day when a tank was opened to enable the patient to receive special care such as physiotherapy. Another necessity was the suctioning of the frequently copious fluids from the throat and windpipe, sometimes requiring a special tube or a bronchoscope.

An unusual twist took place during the polio experience, especially at its height. My perception was that the majority of the doctors working at the Isolation Hospital in our team effort did so without direct remuneration. Most of us were in private practice. Some of us had partners (as I did) or clinics who supported us. The challenge of overcoming or just coping with the epidemic ravishing our extended community, was uppermost in our minds. Working together, the new teams of doctors and nurses kept many patients alive for days, weeks, and a few of them now up to thirty-six years.

With the demands of the new machines, supplies, and unusual equipment, Norman Stanners and Bob Rawlings, the RAH engineer and electrician, were on call day and night for weeks. During the initial days of working with the iron lungs, it was realized that there was a dangerous potential for a leak developing somewhere in the system, allowing the pressure in the tank to fall. The patient would not be able to call for help. By good luck I had a clever neighbour across the street, Ed Adams, who owned a small instrument company. Experimenting with the tub of an old washing machine, he devised a fail-safe alarm and installed one on the top of each respirator.

In the event of an electrical failure, there was, in addition to a flashlight, a three-foot iron bar under each tank. This could be quickly attached and the bellows pumped by hand. One memorable evening, during an electrical storm, the whole hospital went dark just after seven o'clock. Students from the nurses' residence "instinctively" ran across the yard to give assistance, dressed in slacks or whatever. Not a single patient in the nineteen respirators died. The next day a big diesel-electric generator was installed in the yard next to the building, ready to supply standby power within eight seconds.

Monitoring the patient's condition was primitive by today's standards. The individual charts were moved out of the nurses' station to the side of the patient. Flow sheets and graphs were designed and adopted. Some of these resembled operating room records. Much more frequent readings of pulse rate, blood pressure, temperature, and traditional clinical signs became a necessity. An electrocardiogram was available only upon special request from the laboratory. Tests for biochemistry at this time were rudimentary but helped. But the analysis of blood gases which are so important and are taken for granted today, were not available to us.

Dr. George Elliott enlisted the help of Dr. Harold V. Rice, then professor of physiology in the Faculty of Medicine. Although not a medical doctor until later, Harold quickly became interested in our problems. In his lab he devised a portable Van Slyke type of apparatus which could be used in our wards to determine the carbon dioxide concentration in the patient's expelled air. This was a god-send, because before this we could only estimate the proper settings of rate and volume of the respirator. The normal body regulates the proportions of blood gases by adjusting the heart and breathing rates. Harold also donated many hours on the wards and in 1955 published a clinical paper centered on the epidemic.

Drs. Ludvig Sherman, Ted Aaron, and many Edmonton physicians also made significant contributions. Surgeons Colin Dafoe, Colin Ross, Jack Lees, and Ken Clarke performed the bulk of over one hundred and fifty tracheostomies in a make-shift operating room. Dr. Ted Gain of the University Hospital was one of several anaesthetists who took turns in the wards and the operating room for a week or more. Alastair MacKay took daytime duty full time for several weeks to help provide needed continuity. Very few Edmonton physicians declined to serve in the polio wards. But scores of women and men in various ways gave willing and outstanding help, sacrificing time from their usual occupations or jobs, their families, and their leisure. The women's auxiliary of the RAH made an exceptionally strong contribution of money and time toward the physical and mental comfort of the patients.

In the last days of November, my father died in the Royal Alexandra Hospital after a short illness. I was uncomfortable with the realization that I was not paying enough attention to our beloved parents. Priorities at that time were uncertain. One afternoon I went home to have supper with my wife and family, looking forward to a good night's rest. I had an unaccustomed headache, a sore throat, and sore neck. As the evening wore on my anxiety increased, as I knew that these were among the early symptoms of polio. By noon the next day I felt well enough to realize that my fears were groundless.

One of the many duties faced by nurses and doctors

was the need to make empathetic communication, not only with our patients, but with their parents and close relatives. Visitors were not allowed in the wards of those in the acute phases of the disease. Of course this was agonizing for all, especially for children. I believe that the isolation regime contributed to more emotional involvement of staff members. Russell Taylor's leadership and enthusiasm and good sense was a steadying influence.

We also experienced emotional lifts. The best were naturally the clinical successes, when formerly critically-ill patients were sent on to convalescent and rehabilitation facilities, and for physiotherapy, speech therapy and other support services. We were more than happy to pass on our respirator patients to the capable care of specially-trained doctors and supporting staff at the University of Alberta Hospital. Dr. Brian Sproule was one of those who were outstanding in the care of both the acute and the chronic problems.

The weeks and months of coping with this prominent and memorable epidemic have, thankfully, not recurred. Between July 1953 and to March 1954, 415 patients were admitted to the Royal Alexandra Hospital with the diagnosis of poliomyelitis, 43 of whom died. Practically 25 percent required a respirator. Many of the survivors received on-going supportive therapy and continuing care in the excellent facilities developed in the University of Alberta Hospital. The polio vaccines that were produced in the mid-1950s soon reduced new outbreaks to a minimum. The disease still occurs sporadically but mostly in developing countries. And now, some thirty or more years later, a new phenomenon has been reported called the "post-polio syndrome," in which some previously paralysed patients develop a recurrence of severe fatigue, weakness, and pain. Some now require crutches or even a wheelchair.

Looking back at this time, the medical community of Edmonton and of central Alberta, with the cooperation of hospital and of provincial authorities, assembled, staffed, and directed what was probably the first intensive care facility in this part of Canada. One could speculate that the wartime service of many of the men and women involved helped to organize and sustain that innovative medical effort as rapidly as it did.

CHAPTER THREE

Breathing and Bravery

J.F. Elliott, MD

Memories of the Alberta Polio Epidemic 1953-54

Infantile paralysis! We did know something about that disease. Its official name was acute anterior poliomyelitis and it was caused by a virus that attacked the anterior horn cells of the spinal cord. There were two subtypes, or was it three? It was a disease of infants and children which often resulted in muscle weakness and atrophy. The patients were cared for by the orthopedic surgeons. They supervised the Provincial Special Unit at the University Hospital. It was they who gave the lectures about this disease to medical students.

But *this* disease in 1953 was not "infantile paralysis." It was *something else*. It was not infantile — most of the patients were young adults "in the prime of life," although a few children were affected. It *was* paralysis — but it also spread rapidly to the brain and produced paralysis of the centres for swallowing and breathing and

45

sometimes other cranial nerves. It was life-threatening and too often fatal, and its incidence reached epidemic proportions. We had never seen this before. I had not even read about it. To us, it was a new disease. Our lack of knowledge was only exceeded by our lack of equipment and facilities for treatment and, at first, a lack of staff.

Like a war or a tornado, it was hell to live with; but like those disasters, it inspired many among patients' relatives, friends, attendants, nurses, and doctors to deeds of sacrifice and bravery.

Thirty-six years have now gone by. Some of us have been asked many times to write about it — for the archives, for the college, and for the record. I know that the memories stirred up after long conscious neglect may be blurred and distorted, but I hope the main outlines are true. I also hope that the associated emotions have been muted by the passage of time.

This is a personal account, not a scientific paper, not figures, not physiology, not statistics, not pathology, but memories of people; people sick, people dying, people helping people through self-sacrifice and service with no thought of reward.

The site of action was the isolation unit of the Royal Alexandra Hospital, always a dismal place — a "pest house" — now demolished.

I was a latecomer on the scene. My first contact was on a Saturday afternoon when my partner asked me if I would see a patient of his, recently admitted to the Isolation Ward. I found that the patient was in a respirator (an iron lung) and was deemed to be doing all right as were the other eight to ten patients. All were under the medical care of two doctors who looked exhausted.

Later I found the sequence of events had been as follows:

One of the early polio admissions was the son of a member of the Department of Anesthesia at the Royal Alexandra Hospital, Dr. Nelson Nix. He had been admitted because of difficulty in swallowing and breathing. His father, with his training in respiratory function and control, was staying in the building or at least close by. When the nursing staff had problems with similar patients they found him available and asked his advice. He usually contacted the patient's doctor for approval to supervise his patient. This offer was usually gratefully accepted. Who could give better care of failing respiration that one trained in anesthesia?

Next, a general practitioner from the Allin Clinic, Dr. Russ Taylor, had seen that help was needed for 24-hour coverage of an increasing number of critically ill patients in respirators. He had volunteered his services and in preparation had gone to Minneapolis for two weeks to observe their polio care. I believe that Sister Kenny was in Minneapolis at that time and her methods of treatment had been widely reported. On his return, Dr. Taylor worked full time, and I mean full time, in the unit with Dr. Nix. The Allin Clinic gave their approval and their staff cared for his patients.

More medical staff was obviously needed, the two attending physicians being extremely fatigued. I asked if I could help. I was somewhat surprised and puzzled by their negative reactions — how much time could I spend? I offered one afternoon, one day a week, three days a week, with always the same answer — that wouldn't really help much. Full time with the unit? "That might help." I checked with my partner, Dr. John Scott, and he, of course, agreed and took over my medical practice.

What about my wife and three small children? There was no vaccine. The disease was reaching epidemic proportions and people were dying from it. My wife, being her own dedicated self and a former nurse, agreed with me at once, insisting only that I undress in the back porch and have a tub bath and change of clothes, ensuring that my "polio clothes" were hung on a clothes-line in the backyard, before I had any contact with the children. She and they saw little of me for the next couple of months. One son tells me that I was so tired that I would sometimes start to read and go to sleep on the chesterfield.

I soon learned why my working a few hours a day, or a few days a week would have helped little and would have even been an extra burden at first. Nelson and Russ didn't have any time or energy for extra burdens.

I had to be taught how to diagnose polio and exclude other diseases. I learned that the spinal fluid might be normal at the onset, and might show polymorphs early, not the lymphocytes I expected. I had to know when a respirator was needed, when to do a trach, how to get a patient comfortably (?) settled down in a respirator complete with catheter, intravenous, blood pressure cuff, and often tracheostomy and nasogastric tube. The neck piece had to be airtight and all manipulations had to be done through the port holes on the side of the respirator.

I had to be taught to manipulate the respirators. A wrong sequence of procedure could bend the front piece and result in a loss of the vacuum so that the patient would have to be moved to, and established in a new machine. The damaged one would be out of commission until repaired.

And the medical care of patients was complex.

Of first importance was the supervision of respiration. Arterial blood gases were to come much later. We didn't even have a vitalometer, so we depended on checking and recording of pulse rate, blood pressure, color, and general condition — crude monitors all. Occasionally coma or convulsions occurred and sometimes we could not be certain if they were due to hypoxia, CO_2 retention, or hyperventilation. Then care of tracheostomy tubes, fluid, nutrition, bowels, skin etc., etc., etc.

Bronchoscopies were needed. There was no humidification and with a tracheotomy, crusts frequently formed in the trachea and bronchi. These often produced areas of pulmonary atelectasis (collapse of part of the lung). When these were troublesome, removal through a bronchoscope was often carried out. Sometimes these were performed by Dr. Ken Clarke, an Ears, Nose and Throat (ENT) specialist who came in daily. He did a great number of tracheostomies, but often our own staff did the bronchoscopies. I remember one day we got a new bronchoscope, having not had a useful one for a day or two. Dr. Clarke bronchoscoped a husky young farm lad, who had not had a tracheostomy. The patient bit down hard, crushed and bent the bronchoscope as well as taking a nip out of Dr. Clarke's finger. So another bronchoscope was required. I won't repeat Dr. Clarke's comments. Incidentally, this patient has been under my care and still needs a rocking bed or chest respirator. He is married and has a van in which he and his wife travel the country. They have recently moved into a new housing unit especially designed for disabled persons.

Circumstances forced the birth of a new concept in patient care. It became obvious that putting a patient in a respirator in a private room, even with a special nurse who, of course, didn't know any more and perhaps less about his care than we did, was dangerous and sometimes fatal, so all patients (men and women) in tank respirators were put in one big room under constant supervision of the circulating staff. It also was soon obvious that having the charts in an office was useless and the chart of each patient went on his respirator. Dr. Taylor pointed out that this was really Alberta's first Intensive Care Unit. Much later and more deliberately, Dr. Taylor established another intensive care unit at the University Hospital — the Coronary Care Unit.

As we learned from the situation, we also learned from the patients. One of the many things we learned from some of our patients was "frog breathing." It was noted that some patients, when out of the respirator for a short time, would make gulping and swallowing movements. At first we tried to discourage such nonsense, but soon found that some patients could maintain adequate respiratory exchange at least for short periods by collecting air in the mouth and then forcing it into the lungs by a swallowing movement. Some of the patients are still depending, at least in part, on this method when awake.

In those desperate times, doctors pulled together and learned from one another. To my knowledge, during this acute epidemic, payment to doctors was never mentioned, considered, or given, something that should perhaps be more widely known in these days of concern and criticism of doctor's salaries and fee schedules. When the need was there, the medical profession willingly and freely did all they could without thought of financial reward. Many doctors came and worked in the unit. Each brought his unique perspective, his particular strength and expertise. I remember especially Dr. Andrew Cairns, who had the knack of making a patient comfortable in a respirator, adjusting neck pieces, changing positions, raising or lowering the head; Dr. Sproule, whose interest in things pulmonary may have begun at this time; Dr. Kidd spent an afternoon with one of our problem cases who had episodes of convulsions and loss of consciousness, sometimes being over-ventilated and sometimes hypoxic without change in the rate of his iron lung. Dr. Kidd found that he was doing some breathing on his own; enough that if he breathed with the respirator, he would be hyperventilated and if he breathed against it, he would become hypoxic. He was readily controlled when his own respiration was paralysed with curare.

We had psychiatric help too. About all a patient in a respirator with a "trach" could do was roll the eyes, chew, and spit. The spitting was a common reaction. This sometimes upset the nurses. The psychiatrists told us that their main job was to help the nurses adjust to any unusual or negative reaction of the patients. On one occasion, an orthopedic surgeon was assessing the degree of muscle loss. He took the patient out of the respirator and started his examination before realizing that the patient couldn't breathe. Someone came and did the bagging before he got too hypoxic. At one stage, if I recall correctly, Dr. John Scott took the then Premier Ernest Manning to the isolation unit to show him the extent and the difficulties of the epidemic. The Premier did what he could to expedite supplies and arranged for the construction of a new wing on the south end of the University Hospital called the "polio wing." It still stands though it is not being used, except by occasional flocks of pigeons.

Doctors represented only one part of the outpouring of commitment that came unfailingly and ungrudgingly from all levels of staff and from the general public. More nurses were needed at first. Then came hardy volunteers who took the risks and did yeoman service in a difficult and dangerous environment. Some, understandably, didn't come because of risk to children and husbands at home.

Some care necessitated removal of patients from respirators. How to care for patients in tank respirators? They still needed skin care, and often catheters, enemas, intravenous lines, and a variety of other procedures. The Edmonton Academy of Medicine came to the rescue and organized teams of doctors who visited daily and "bagged" patients i.e. gave artificial respiration with manual compression of a rubber bag allowing removal from the tank respirators for necessary care. This went on for months. They also organized rotations of volunteer sleep-in doctors to cover night emergencies. One of the volunteers was Dr. Donovan Ross, the then Minister of Health for Alberta.

Life was strenuous. Life was exciting. Life was depressing. Hours were long, deaths were frequent, often with progressive hyperthermia or hypotension which could not be controlled even with massive doses of Laevophed — sometimes with aspiration, so doing a tracheostomy became almost routine for patients going into respirators. Many had gastrointestinal hemorrhages from peptic ulcers. There was gamma globulin, in limited supply, to be used for children (and pregnant mothers) who were exposed. I remember going to the house of a mother with two small children and giving the gamma globulin to the two children. The mother wasn't pregnant so she couldn't have it. The children stayed well, but the mother developed a complete limb and respiratory paralysis without really having a fever or being otherwise ill. She did recover. When the supply was adequate, the staff took occasional injections of the gamma globulin, especially if one had a headache and a bit of neck stiffness.

Not all the tragedies occurred in hospital. A plane from Grande Prairie carrying a doctor and polio patient to our unit disappeared and the wreckage was not found for many months. Dr. Ted Bell, in charge of the University Hospital laboratories, developed a transverse myelitis — probably a variant of the same disease, and remained paralyzed from the waist down. When over the acute phase, he carried on and ran an outstanding laboratory from his wheelchair.

Some of us became so involved that for days and sometimes nights too, our minds and bodies were completely occupied concerning the care of patients in the unit. For myself, after a time, if someone contacted me about his or her illness, if he or she could still breathe normally, I could not really accept that their illness was severe or needing emergency treatment. *How narrow one's interests can become!* On one occasion, I was reprimanded by some of my family. I was asked to see a nurse in bed in the University Hospital, to say whether she had polio. She did, with one weak leg and I so reported. Only afterwards did I learn that she was my first cousin whom I knew when in her nurse's uniform but did not recognize when she was ill and in bed. There is a story about not recognizing a patient with her

54

clothes on — this time I didn't recognize her with her clothes off! My tour of duty in the unit ended when my friends and family decided my health was suffering. The rate of admissions had settled down and everyone had time to sleep. My wife and I went on a much appreciated holiday to Hana on Maui in Hawaii. We could afford the rates at the time!

Convalescence and chronic care came after the acute illness was over and stabilized. This meant further equipment: wheel chairs, physiotherapy, etc., again much of it outside of our realm of expertise. We were fortunate to obtain an enthusiastic young physiatrist, Michael Carpendale, who came to the University Hospital and supervised rehabilitation. Unfortunately for us, he stayed only a couple of years.

Arrangements were made for transfer from the isolation unit at the Royal Alexandra Hospital to other hospitals, mainly the University. It became obvious that "total care" was needed and there was a weekly meeting of all concerned to revise and advise on each case. The members included: an internist, physiatrist, orthopaedic surgeon, social worker, and sometimes a psychiatrist. This was the first "team conference" for total care with which I was involved. It is now being found necessary for the care of the elderly. It taught me that the physician is only one member of the team of health care specialists, although he may, sometimes, be the quarterback.

In retrospect, I believe the polio epidemic resulted in an intensive care unit (the first in Alberta?) and later in the concept of comprehensive care by many members of different branches of medical services working as a team.

Postscript

From time to time during the polio epidemic and in the first days of its abatement, discussion arose about the heroics of saving a patient destined for complete paralysis and life in a respirator (the old ethics problem). Those of us who worked in the unit had seen patients almost completely paralyzed, who had almost complete recovery, and had no doubt about doing all we could. However, we didn't think those who remained severely paralyzed and required respiratory assistance would survive for long. We thought complications such as infections and kidney stones would occur and bring death in a few years. How wrong we were. In the fall of 1987 the survivors held a party at Rundle Park. Dr. Taylor, Dr. Sproule, and I attended. We were just amazed at the accomplishments as well as the survival of the severely paralyzed people. There were about thirty who attended. What *willpower, determination,* and *sheer guts* can accomplish!

Dr. Taylor expressed it well, saying one didn't know exactly what produced this miraculous survival and accomplishment, but that it was extraordinary power that was present (he had a lot of that too). I am still amazed at the survival and accomplishments of the respiratory polio patients, but I thank Heaven for the Salk and Sabin vaccines, which should prevent any recurrence of such an epidemic!

CHAPTER FOUR

Poliomyelitis

B.J. Sproule, MD

Poliomyelitis is an infectious disease of the nervous system — the last epidemic of which occurred at a time when a biologic approach to medicine was emerging. The sudden catastrophic appearance of dozens of patients unable to breathe and requiring assistance, was an impetus that accelerated the development of physiologic measurements of lung function, of respiratory therapy departments, of air ambulance services, and of critical care units.

All of these developments encompassed a scientific biologic approach. Interlaced with, and as a background to these, however, were the humane qualities of kindness and sympathy inherent in the art of Medicine and hallowed as its priestly function. Such personal compassion is not of course the private preserve of the physician and is shared by many givers of medical care. During the early days of the epidemic that struck Edmonton, these qualities were shown by very many physicians as well as by others. Three physicians particularly should be mentioned: Dr. Russ Taylor, Dr. Frank Elliott, and Dr. Nelson Nix, but many physicians devoted themselves in a selfless way which should inspire us all.

As a consequence of the poliomyelitis epidemic detailed on the previous pages, a number of initiatives were taken from which flowed new programs, and these continue each day to benefit patients with breathing problems.

The epidemic of 1953 was largely handled at the Royal Alexandra Hospital but also by physicians from throughout the city.

A smaller group of patients was cared for between 1954 and 1957 on St. Mary's ward of the General Hospital. In early 1954 there were only two patients (a nurse and a physician) in the University Hospital.

As has been previously mentioned, it was accepted in those days that a certain proportion of each physician's effort should be given to those in need without expectation of payment. Of some interest, too, in these days of union confrontation, nurses and orderlies frequently worked extra, or secretaries double, shifts without payment or compensating time off, deeming it a privilege to help. Part of this I believe resulted from a sense of rapidly acquired competence, easily achieved then. It is much harder to quickly acquire that comfort level in this age of intimidating technology.

It was in the early dramatic and event-filled days that Dr. Harold Rice, the Chairman of Physiology at the University, urged by Dr Frank Elliott, visited the polio ward and after a cursory glance abandoned the academic confines of the physiology laboratory to hurl himself into this living physiological experiment. The bodies imprisoned in the clanking, sighing tank respirators (Drinkers and Emersons) were inaccessible in their metal cages, but did represent living, dramatic ongoing exercises in pulmonary physiology. The usefulness of the carbon dioxide blood level as an index of the adequacy of ventilation was appreciated by Dr. Rice and led him to construct an apparatus for the evaluation of end–tidal CO_2 (the carbon dioxide level measured in the expired breath at the end of a breath out) as an index of effective ventilation. Unexpected disparities between "guestimated" and actual ventilation resulted in adjustments in the pressure or rates of the ventilator and produced improvements in blood pressure and pulse of the patients and the transformation of grey, clammy, agitated, or semi–stuporous faces protruding from the foam collars at the end of the tank ventilator to faces of tranquility and ruddy vigor. The air conditioning and humidifying action of the nose and upper airway on lower airway function was only dimly perceived at this time. Patients with open tracheostomies were then being subjected to repetitive ramming of a traumatizing rigid bronchoscope into the airways to remove rapidly-accumulating encrusted and inspissated secretions. The cautious use of homemade humidifying devices over the open tracheostomy sites and then the tentative trickling of drops of saline directly into the lung, which in turn was followed by increasingly more vigorous flushing of the tracheal bronchial tree with a few hundred millilitres of fluid effectively obviated this problem. The use of humidifiers on our bone-dry western Canadian wards is still of importance for patients functioning in the parched atmosphere found inside during a western Canadian winter.

I was impressed by the dramatic demonstration of the utility of CO_2 assessment and as a research fellow in Dallas, Texas a year or two after this, I learned to manipulate a Haldane apparatus, a dropping mercury electrode, the Riley Microbubble syringe (so wonderfully described by Dr. Campbell in *Not Always on the Level*) and, finally, a Clark polarographic electrode.

These numbingly boring activities represented stages in an evolution which has since spawned the bewildering thicket of blood gas numbers which proliferate on charts in all major hospitals. It is astonishing that these patients on ventilatory assistance survived and sometimes flourished when the only guide to ventilation was Dr. Rice's CO_2 measuring system and "guesstimation" by the physicians. Once back from Dallas I established a crude but reasonably effective polarographic system for measuring blood gases that simplified matters considerably.

In May 1954 the patients from the other hospitals were transferred to the University Hospital where they have resided since. It was not then clear that this frightening and dreadful disease would be defeated by an effective vaccine. The provincial government therefore committed itself to constructing an extra wing on the

University Hospital (to be called the Polio Wing). From original temporary quarters on a ward of the old University Hospital, all patients were moved in 1956 to a portion of the newly constructed wing. Their numbers were gradually augmented by fifteen victims in 1957, seven in 1958, and then surged in 1959 with thirty-three patients while a mini-epidemic in 1960 added ninety-eight patients, of whom forty-two had received three or more injections of Salk vaccine.

The concept of a "closed" ICU (Intensive Care Unit) with a team approach to patient care and with a single physician "in charge" by rotation, one-on-one around the clock, commenced in embryo form on the Royal Alexandra wards. This approach continued at the University where all patients were assigned to four physicians in rotation (Drs. Elliott, Fraser, Aaron, and Dvorkin) and, with reactions ranging from boundless confidence to naked fear, members of the staff formed a roster for emergency care of these patients at night.

I joined this staff (as a medical resident) at the same time as did surgical resident, Dr. Alvin Mooney. We were given a sleeping room to share on the ward, a small stipend, and the opportunity to cover any emergencies. Fringe benefits included unlimited access to toast and tea and conversation with the nurses (leading possibly to my courtship and marriage with the supervisor, Marnie McKay).

The physiotherapists became more knowledgeable about breathing as they wrestled with the problems of moving limbs while hampered by the cumbersome tank ventilators. Dietitians regularly agonized over appropriate blends and techniques that might be used to feed the patients with bulbar palsy. Psycho-emotional difficulties and interfamily relationships were explored by the staff and a few social workers. In short, the skeleton of a comprehensive ICU was assembled for subsequent fleshing out. Breathing during the initial epidemic was accomplished in the tank respirators supplanted by hand bagging of patients as they were bathed and moved. At times of power failure the instant mobilization of all categories of staff and visitors to pump anesthetic bags was awesome. The potential importance of lung collapse and stiffening when mechanical breaths were provided at a fixed tidal volume was recognized and tanks were periodically "vacuumed," the forerunner of distending airway pressure as a supportive modality. This also involved applying a sudden sucking burst of negative pressure to a port in the tank to achieve a bigger breath.

Other kinds of respiratory aid were introduced and, as a resident, I was the first to try out a rocking bed we received. Thirty-five minutes of rocking produced, to my own humiliation but to the obvious delight of observers, an extremely impressive and explosive emesis.

A Haliburton positive pressure ventilator, a water bath, some tubing, and the controls for a Clark polarographic electrode were part of the Dallas legacy (which also included four children hatched under the hot Texas sun). The positive pressure ventilator was applied during one long night to a freshly tracheotomized polio patient. Effective ventilation was achieved with remarkable ease. Inspired air was completely humidified. The pulse, chest, abdomen, and all body parts were accessible for assessment and care. This represented significant improvement over the groping and fumbling which went on through the ports of the tank ventilator. It became increasingly obvious that there were a variety of other patients who were breathing poorly, ineffectively, or not at all (cervical, spinal injuries, pneumonias, etc.) who could be managed by a positive pressure ventilator and ventilated on an ordinary ward. They, however, by necessity required around the clock nursing if they were to be managed in any sort of acceptable manner. Fairly soon it seemed sensible for such victims to be grouped together in a four-bedded ward. Thus, one-on-one nursing could be co-ordinated with the other professional activities, at first provided by the disorganized efforts of attending physicians and residents, and then incrementally by increasingly more capable respiratory therapists and physiotherapists. Our activities continued in this manner for quite some time, and then the whole operation took a giant leap forward when Dr. Garner King returned from training in Denver. We made representation to Hospital Administration which led to the carving out of space for a six-bedded ICU on one of the large open wards in the old 1912 wing of the hospital. Within a year or two, further agitation led to a second move into quarters previously occupied by the polio patients who had been moved to the Aberhart Hospital. This left the original six beds to become the Burn Unit of the hospital. The Aberhart Hospital, originally a TB Sanatorium, has gradually added other functions so that it now has Respiratory, Polio, Auxiliary, and Rehabilitation beds in addition to a continued responsibility for tuberculosis.

For a period of time the IPPB (intermittent positive pressure breathing) machine was perceived to be not only a useful instrument for ventilating paralysed people, but a panacea for all lung ailments. Out-patient treatments and "puff parlours" attained a brief burst of popularity. We never did use out-patient treatments to any extent, but our hospital did acquire an impressive forest of IPPB machines used largely for the delivery of bronchodilator medications and requiring a good deal of care and feeding. It now is considered to be tantamount to malpractice to use such a machine for merely delivering mist but, if available, I believe there may still be a distinct role for them in some unco-ordinated and unco-operative patients.

Our first respiratory therapists were myself and the residents and we were able to destroy or make non-functioning breathing machines about as rapidly as we were able to put the blood gas apparatus out of commission. Although frequently non-operative, the blood gas machine that I assembled did acquire increasing favour. At that time too, valiant attempts were made to personally use or to persuade residents and students to use Moran Campbell's rebreathing CO_2 technique for monitoring CO_2 on the ward, but I never succeeded in making this a routine. Our first full-time respiratory therapist was from Montreal, more or less self-taught as all of us were then. He started servicing equipment in a dark corner next to the furnace in the sub-basement of the hospital. The stygian darkness was reminiscent of the sewers of Paris with the steady drip of condensate from the ceiling contributing to difficulties in keeping the equipment from rusting. He, however, had a great penchant for administration and for pulling the necessary administrative levers and we fairly quickly managed to move from the sub-basement to the basement and into an area with a desk and a few pale shafts of sunlight. A succession of terrific, trained-on-the-job, practical, caring as well as mechanically adept orderlies manned the "Department of Inhalation Therapy" as it gradually developed. Les Gado, a particularly compassionate and knowledgeable orderly, was one such forerunner of respiratory therapists.

Progress of another order of magnitude then occurred when an academic program was started at the Northern Alberta Institute of Technology some twenty years ago. It has now evolved so that individuals with the Two Year Program as a base are administrators at higher levels in government and in hospital hierarchies, and competition to enter the program has become fierce. Graduates with a variety of university degrees compete with superior high school graduates for positions in the program. With a background in respiratory therapy, graduates can and frequently do move into other technical areas in the health system such as pulmonary function laboratories, catheterization, research labs, and so forth. Recent years have seen the development of post-graduate programs and of augmented training and it appears likely that before long University programs with Masters' degrees in some of the subdisciplines of inhalation therapy will be developed.

Respiratory Home Care also originated in the poliomyelitis ward and was, here in Edmonton, an outgrowth of this epidemic. In the first days a few determined patients with brave and dedicated attendants would go home on weekends despite the voiced fierce opposition and protestations of those more prudent.

Five of the original patients had polio insurance of $5,000 each which, when augmented by funds from the March of Dimes Polio Foundation (managed by the Canadian Legion), provided equipment and personnel support for them to move home permanently utilizing housekeeping and orderly assistance. In those days the Polio Foundation collected in their drives about $250,000-$500,000 per year in Alberta. Dr. Frank Elliott, as Chairman of the Hospital Polio Committee, pressed successfully for capital purchases of homecare equipment by government. The maintenance and upkeep of wheelchairs, rocking beds, and so forth as well as some personnel assistance was then provided by the Polio Foundation.

An ancillary benefit was that in developing proposals to National Health and Welfare for funding for equipment for a lung function laboratory, a persuasive argument seemed to be that measurements of lung volume and mechanics and diffusing capacity were essential if one was to adequately assess this group for a trial of care at home. Blood gas equipment had been accepted already as essential for monitoring these paralysed people and some studies done on patients with fractures and fat embolism further underlined the possibility of assessing oxygenation in other disease states.

In 1967, after much representation, it was agreed that the University Hospital (at the Aberhart site) under a separate budget, would provide respiratory therapy services to hospitalized patients with chronic lung disease and a Chronic Respiratory Support Ward was developed and on the same floor as the Polio Ward. In 1974 support was obtained for a three-year pilot project of Respiratory Home Care involving the provision of equipment and regular home visitation by a team of nurses, physiotherapists, respiratory therapists, and the occasional social worker. All team members were encouraged to have interchangeable skills and, if necessary, to function in other roles. As was the wont of pilot projects, it grew invisibly and became quietly incorporated into the global budget of the hospital and is now an established part of the operation capably directed by Dr Neil Brown. There has been a certain amount of triumph and self-satisfaction about achieving this progress but it was probably related to administrative torpor as much as to fiery advocacy. It was possible to slip programs into the administrative maw where they became gelatinously adherent and were gradually accepted as part of the essential order. Now, of course, in this era of evaluation, re-evaluation, and paper justification (all unquestionably laudable), the development of programs in this manner will be more difficult and I have a fear that we may miss some possibilities.

The Respiratory Home Care group now provides comprehensive support for 220 patients or "clients" to use a term I still abhor. The majority of us, whether termed patients or clients, and depending upon the support structure, can manage better functionally and socially in a home environment and this can in turn usually be provided more economically.

As an outgrowth, therefore, of the poliomyelitis epidemic in the early 1950s, impetus was given to the development of the number of interrelated respiratory programs. The beginnings of the Intensive Care Units, air ambulance, inhalation therapy, respiratory therapy, respiratory home care, and a pulmonary function laboratory all occurred in those traumatic and event-filled days.

a poem for clayton may's memorial service

young lads
excited
growing

full of the
  vitality
    exuberance
    and vigor

that characterizes
  childhood

the strong
  muscles
    sinews
    and nerves
  running
  jumping
  pushing

  exploring
the limits
  of their
    strength
    and endurance

their growth
and development
a seemingly
limitless
horizon
of movement
and dexterity

full of the
promise
of manhood
and
maturity

into these
peaceful
surroundings
of home
and village

came a prairie
plague

borne somehow
on the
summer storm
in the
august
heat

like an
ancient
scythe

it chose
to harvest
the young
and
the strong

paralysis

infantile

dark
mysterious
foreboding

where once
there had
been
steady
measured

breathing

there was
now
short
anxious
rapid
pants

gasping
pleading

for air
for breath
for life

but
for hundreds
there was in
the night
only

one
long breath

that ended
in
silence

the muscles
voluntary
and involuntary

alive
but
dead

unresponsive
to the
minute
electrical
impulses

that called
for
movement
and
action

iron lung
the boldly
crude
attempt
to
overcome
paralysis

mechanical
miracle

such a simple

life giving

prison

today
  three and
    one-half
    decades
      later

a man
  is buried

after a
  summer storm
  under
    a cloudless
    sky

he had once been a
  boy

    who ran
    and
      skipped

    as young
      boys do

but somehow
  he was
    marked

    to suffer

in that
  prison

paralyzed

what marks a

  man
  as a
    man

what he does
  what he says

his exercise
  of power

the accumulation
  of wealth

the service of his
  fellowman

    these and
    more

in the life
  and times

    of

  clayton

we know
  in our hearts

  that we have
  witnessed
  again

the greatness
  of the
    human
      spirit

hidden
  in a
  deformed
    ravaged
      body

a gift was
  given to the world
    in his
      birth

a greater gift
    was given
      to us
  in his
      living

a poem
  and tribute

written to
memorialize
the life and death

of clayton

  july 1988

      r

Vignettes

I believe that it was on a September morning that I was called in the main OR (operating room) to take an urgent message from the Isolation. A young boy had just arrived with breathing trouble. Grasping my tracheal intubation basket I hurried five flights down the back stairwell, not waiting for an elevator. He was lying in the admitting room across the yard, gasping and nearly black. It was easy to put the breathing tube in place as he was so weak, and in a few minutes his color turned to blessed pink with 100 percent oxygen. This boy's breathing muscles were only slightly affected but the throat and voice box never regained their normal function. He learned to talk by closing the opening in his neck with a finger-tip. With this disability but with tremendous will he finished school, graduated from the University of Alberta, and became a successful professional.

— Dr. N. Nix —

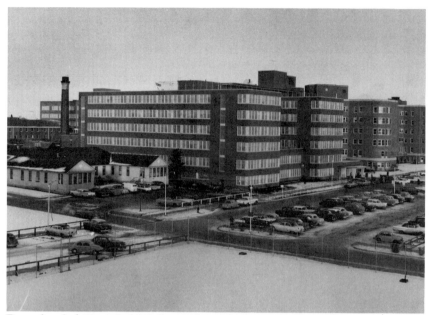

Provincial Special Unit and main hospital (right). Later the first Provincial Cancer Clinic, (*Media Services, UAH*).

One of the fairly early problem cases involved a young adult whose paralysis was incomplete but severe enough to require a tank respirator. His skin and lips were blue and there were jerky movements of his limbs and body. This unusual lack of accommodation to the assisted breathing puzzled us, and the University neurology expert of that time predicted dire results because of apparent involvement of the brain. Not wanting to concede defeat, our experience and knowledge of anaesthesia techniques led us to try to test the effect of increasing the depth of paralysis by temporarily administering a drug from our OR supplies. The idea worked. The twitching stopped, the color became normal, and the respirator could do its duty unopposed. We continued the drug slowly, intravenously, over a few days. His own breathing muscles fortunately gradually recovered and he could breathe well on his own. The neck and throat remained weak, but he was allowed to return home after a few weeks.

About two years later I was in my McLeod Building office when the receptionist said "a policeman" in uniform wanted to speak to me. He identified himself to me as the man in the iron lung described above. He had been re-hired by the Edmonton Fire Department as a building inspector. He was fully recovered but needed to wear a neck brace. This man wanted to thank me for helping him to recover. While in the respirator he was conscious and remembered hearing my name. He recalled that at the time he didn't care for me much,

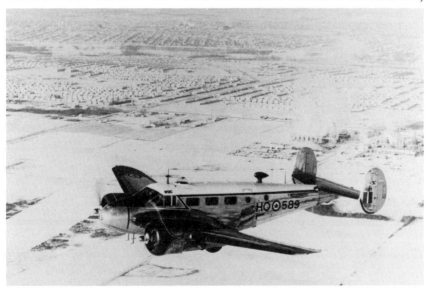

418 Squadron RCAF Beachcraft (C45) with astrodome for star-shots (astral-navigation) as used for rescue flights out of Edmonton, circa 1953-54 (*Dept. Nat. Defence, Ottawa*)

because of his inability to talk or to protest about the situation or the needles. But he later changed his mind, he said.

Our use of the curare-like drug in 1953 in the polio ward was not a discovery by itself, but rather an alternative way to meet an urgent need using a method with which we were familiar in the OR.

— Dr. N. Nix —

One afternoon Dr. Gordon Bell phoned me at the Hospital from a home near the University. He said a

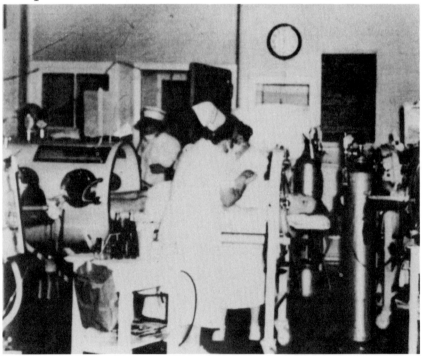

Polio Ward — Isolation Hospital, Royal Alexandra Hospital (from "Under the Flight Path," Royal Alexandra Hospital Nurses Alumni)

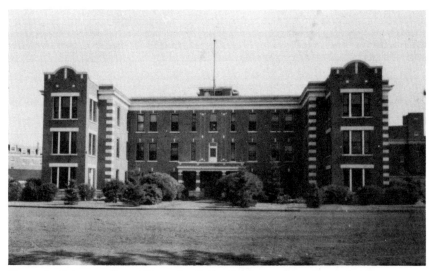

Royal Alexandra Hospital Isolation Annexe (*Edmonton Archives*)

mother with severe breathing problems was on the way by ambulance. Her husband was with her. There was just time to get some equipment before the vehicle was at the door. The urgency was obvious as the man was giving his wife mouth-to-mouth resuscitation. It took only a couple of seconds to get on board, insert a tracheal tube, and pump in oxygen with a breathing bag. Her color and consciousness slowly returned as she was wheeled through the halls and upstairs to the ward. Her husband stayed day and night, attentive and anxious. About the second day he bought a lampshade and installed it above the iron lung to shield his wife's eyes as she lay helpless below. A few days later he became a victim himself, and the two were in ventilators side by side. Unfortunately, however, he must have had a

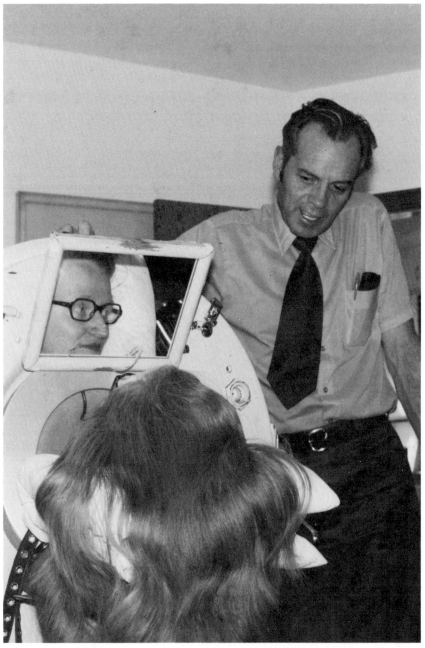

**Dr. Russell Taylor with Connie Kowalski Clark at Norrie
Bishop's house, in Norrie's iron lung**

massive invasion of the virus and the young lawyer died ten days after his wife was admitted.

His wife survived with prolonged hospitalization. About 1957-58 she was allowed to return to her home, with nursing help, oxygen, and a rocking bed especially for sleeping. An infection such as a cold meant return to the hospital and the iron lung for a short period. Despite widespread paralysis and a permanent tracheostomy hole in the windpipe, she learned to speak using her "esophageal voice," with which she would swallow mouthfuls of air and using this air would form understandable words. For several seasons the Edmonton Doctors' Curling League hired her as a telephone secretary. She was able to be at home with her children for several years. During this period, Russ Taylor, keeping in touch in his characteristic selfless way, took her with a ventilator and her housekeeper for a holiday in the Caribbean. Her determination to survive and her incredible cheerfulness impressed everyone. She died in February 1977.

— Dr. N. Nix —

As the epidemic progressed, the staffs at the city hospitals received increasing numbers of calls from rural areas asking for advice and assistance. Clinics and workshops were offered at the Royal Alexandra Hospital for nurses and doctors. Respiratory paralysis was an especially frightful challenge away from the larger centres. There was no organized air-ambulance service. The gravity of the medical emergencies often persuaded the care-givers to undertake risky trips by highway or by air with little regard for the time of day or poor weather. The RCAF Search and Rescue Squadron supplied excellent transportation on many occasions, considering the limited number of airstrips available. Nurses and interns from the city hospitals would be on board when required. Few aircraft at that time had electrical power of 110 volts available to run respirators and suction equipment or monitors. This serious problem was at least partially met by using hand-operated bellows.

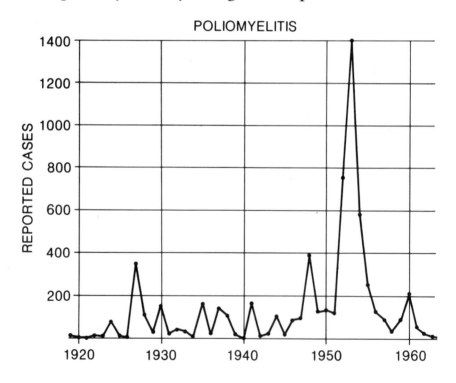

POLIOMYELITIS

On one unforgettable afternoon in late November there was a telephone call from a doctor in Grande Prairie. He had a young man with a serious breathing problem, and said he needed to fly the patient to Edmonton right away. We advised him to wait, if he could, for an aircraft large enough to accommodate a stretcher and with room to administer to necessary treatment on the way. Our team waited late into the evening, but they never did arrive. The wreck of the single-engine Cessna was not found until a year or two later, deep in a forest in the Whitecourt area.

This tragedy affected all of us profoundly. We were haunted with the nagging thoughts of how it might have been prevented if other steps had been taken. The doctor, Donald Broadribb Wilson, a native of the Grande Prairie area, was a 1951 graduate of the University of Alberta. The pilot, Gordon MacDonald, had served four years in the RCAF and was decorated with the Distinguished Flying Cross. These two men gave their lives in a supremely unselfish attempt to save Lloyd Williams. All three young men had families.

— *Dr. N. Nix* —

On another occasion a doctor who had attended one of Russell Taylor's teaching clinics, phoned for help. He had a three-year-old boy alive but unable to breathe on his own. This was in a single-doctor town near the

Saskatchewan border. The problem had kept the small hospital almost totally engrossed for over twenty-four hours. Could we come and get the patient? Dr. Vance MacDonald, a neurosurgeon, offered to accompany me. "Smitty" of Smith's ambulance would drive the four hundred mile round trip largely on gravel roads. We had a small respirator that would work with a spare car battery. The tearful parents were naturally reluctant to see their child go. The return was uneventful until we pulled in for gasoline on the outskirts of Camrose. The station owner refused to refuel the car because of a Wednesday afternoon bylaw, even though I showed him the kid in the respirator through the window. We barely were able to reach the next station down the road.

After several weeks in a respirator this little redhead was making good progress towards recovery, when he died of a cardiac arrest when choking on his supper. I could not control the tears when the nurses called me at home. Even after twelve years of hospital and military service, I was vulnerable to emotion.

— *Dr. N. Nix* —

Early December was the busiest time in the respirator rooms. One evening I was on duty with Dr. Andrew Cairns, another valuable worker from the Allin Clinic. We had thirty-two patients in respirators, a hectic and almost terrifying load. A child of three or four years was admitted with deficient breathing but with good control of his throat. He needed continuous assistance to breathe adequately. But all of our iron lungs had been filled. Almost desperate, I was able to place him in the opposite end of a respirator tank which already contained a child of similar size. There happened to be a service port at the foot end, and we were able to adapt a collar to the child to maintain air pressure in the big

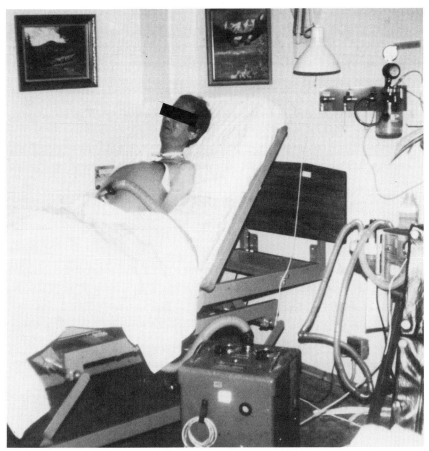

Polio patient on respiratory support with a cuirass (chest piece) ventilator

85

cylinder. This was a questionable procedure of course, and in retrospect it was improper. But the two little ones were carefully monitored during the night and appeared to sleep peacefully and safely. In the morning new equipment arrived, making breathing better for all of us.

On another active night shift, Andrew walked into the respirator ward where I was working. He asked me to come into the adjoining ward because he had been unable to twist open an oxygen cylinder valve. I tried the valve and it seemed to open normally. In a few moments we realized with alarm that Andrew's arm was affected and he was sent off. Incomplete paralysis developed on his left side, but he recovered and was able to return to work in about four months. Three of

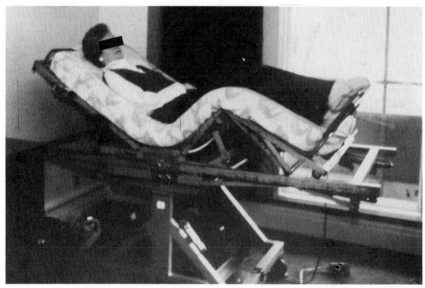

Polio patient on a rocking bed — a device that uses the patient's abdominal contents to move the diaphragms up and down thereby providing ventilation

his children were also affected but fortunately regained their health.

— Dr. N. Nix —

Respirators (Iron Lungs)

The first ones we had, had been donated to Alberta hospitals by Lord Nuffield. They looked for all the world like coffins, but they did work. The next ones were green "Drinker" machines which were much better — proper height, more easily controlled, and with less suggestion of death. Then came a modified Drinker

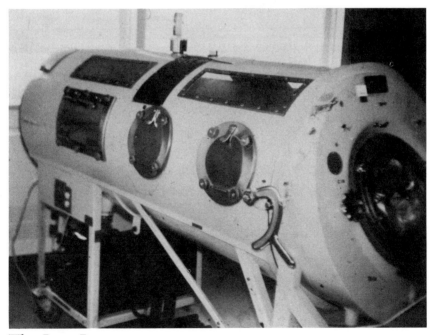

The Iron Lung

87

machine with the front sloped instead of vertical. This helped with procuring a comfortable neck fitting and with the care of trach tubes. Later respirators obtained were big yellow Emersons — more room, easier patient care, and less mechanical trouble.

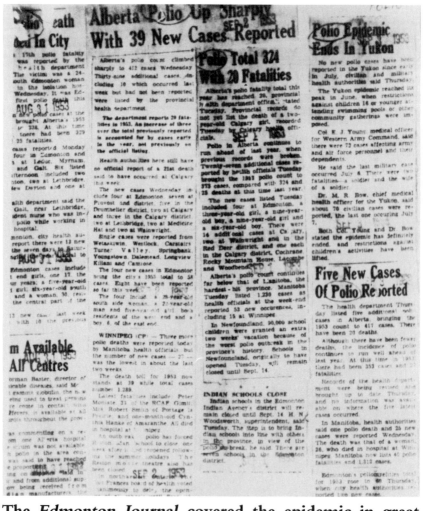

The *Edmonton Journal* covered the epidemic in great detail (*reproduced by permission*)

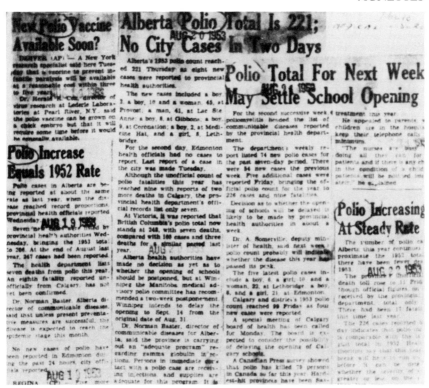

At first, respirators were in short supply. Later adequate numbers were flown in from Winnipeg where there had been an epidemic about two years before.

One day we got a rocking bed. This was an event. The machine had been devised in Saskatoon for the treatment of peripheral vascular disease but was an efficient respiratory aid once the patients became accustomed to it and got over the motion sickness which was common at first.

Several of them are still used by patients in their homes or in auxiliary hospitals. The rocking bed had the great advantage of allowing access to the body of the patient for toileting, skin care, catheterization, or whatever, without having to work through small rubber encased port-holes of the tank respirators.

— *J.F. Elliott* —

In the early 1930s, Lord Nuffield, an English industrialist designed, built, and donated a respirator to every large hospital in the British Empire. The one received by the Edmonton Isolation Hospital was used on and off over the years, but most of the time it was stored in a remote corner covered by a sheet. One of the last patients to use it was Donna Graham, who was struck

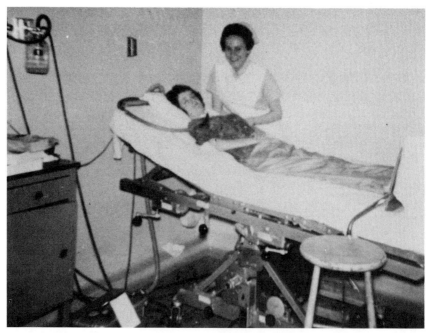

Patient in a rocking bed — Sybil and Miss Holt, June 1961

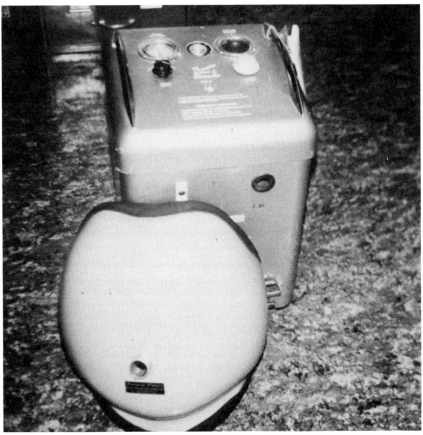

Close up of the chest piece ventilator system

down by polio in March 1953. Donna survived and
became a recognized paint-by-mouth artist. She died
in December 1971.

The Nuffield Respirator was essentially a wooden
box about the size of a coffin on legs. The head of the
patient protruded through an opening in one end, with
a snug rubber collar around the neck to make the tank
air-tight. A pump and bellows underneath made alter-
nating positive and negative pressure in the box. The

91

vacuum phase sucked air into the lungs of the patient, the pressure expelled the air and carbon dioxide. There were windows and portholes in the box through which supportive care could be given, although with some difficulty. Patients were understandably apprehensive. Nursing care was substantially increased and specialized.

Anaesthesiologists were never happy with tank respirators of this sort. Artificial respiration is more efficiently provided by inflating the lungs with positive pressure of air through a face mask or a tube to the lungs. A rubber bag filled with air or oxygen is squeezed by hand or by mechanical means. At the same time, the removal of the waste product carbon dioxide is more efficient.

Metal respirators of the tank type became available and were better than the Nuffield boxes. But in the mid-fifties, research by doctors and engineers was producing totally new respirators using the principle of lung inflation through a tube in the windpipe, using intermittent positive pressure. Much better long-term support for patients who needed sustained artificial breathing resulted. The old iron-lungs were phased out except for special cases.

— *Dr. N. Nix* —

INDEX